Guide to Homeopathic Remedies *for the* Birth Bag

5ᵀᴴ EDITION REVISED

By Patty Brennan

2022 5th Edition Revised
2014 5th Edition
2000 4th Edition
1997 3rd Edition
1990 2nd Edition
1989 1st Edition

Published by Dream Street Press
Ann Arbor, Michigan
Available from LifespanDoulas.com
Manufactured in the United States of America
∞ Printed on acid-free paper

ISBN 978-0-9797247-0-1

Disclaimer
The content of this book is for informational and educational purposes only. The information is not intended to replace professional medical evaluation or advice. The author is not responsible for, and will not be liable for any direct, indirect, consequential, special, exemplary or other damages arising from the use or misuse of any information presented.

Note to the Reader
I am no longer engaged in a clinical practice and do not provide homeopathic consultations, nor give advice via phone or email. Please consider investing in care from a qualified "classical homeopath" in your area.

Dedicated to Patricia Kelly MD, a highly skilled classical homeopath, now (sadly for us) retired. Dr. Kelly provided excellent care to me and my family for many years and I learned a great deal from her. She was a healer with the heart of a teacher and I will be forever grateful.

Acknowledgments

I AM GRATEFUL TO THE FOLLOWING PEOPLE:

My husband and children—Jerry, Terry and Max—who, in faithfully accepting my homeopathic ministrations, have been my greatest teachers over the years.

Pat Kramer, a homebirth midwife pioneer, who modeled resourceful and fearless midwifery, integrated homeopathy into her practice with great success, and co-authored the first edition of this book.

Parvin Panahi, for her excellent design skills and delightful work ethic in turning my booklet into a book.

Preface to the 5th Edition

INCREASING NUMBERS OF CONSUMERS are becoming frustrated with the current medical model of health care. "Side effects" (more accurately described as undesirable drug effects) of many pharmaceuticals have proven to be more dangerous than the problems they were originally designed to cure. Individuals are often treated with several drugs at once, each aimed to counteract symptoms in different parts of the body, and then to counteract symptoms caused by the drugs themselves. In the case of pregnant women, the dangers of drug therapy have been well established. In fact, no drug has been ***proven*** safe for use during pregnancy.

Homeopathy, with its lack of side effects and perfect suitability for home health care, is an excellent choice for both midwives and mothers and, indeed, anyone who works with pregnant, birthing or lactating mothers and their babies. In homeopathy we have a non-toxic, inexpensive, accessible and effective alternative to drug therapy. It is a gentle, holistic modality that incorporates all of the complexities of human beings in the selection of a remedy tailored to the individual. The fact that homeopathy works is evidence of intelligent design in nature. The more one learns, the more amazing it becomes.

This book is designed to simplify selection of the most commonly-indicated remedies for complaints and complications, for mother or baby, during the childbearing year. There are many remedies which are not covered and could, undoubtedly, be called for in some cases. If you are not getting results in a reasonable time frame, given the severity of the presenting symptoms, then consultation with a homeopathic physician or activation of emergency medical care may be warranted. There is no call here for heroic measures at home in place of proper medical care. However, in many cases, such as an infant who is slow to start breathing or a mother who is hemorrhaging, a remedy may be used to stabilize the individual as standard emergency procedures are followed and emergency personnel are called to the scene. It is possible that by the time help arrives, it will no longer be needed, but always err on the side of caution.

In this updated 5th edition, you will find an expanded introduction section for those new to homeopathy and updated resources, as well as additional tips and tools designed to help you quickly select the most appropriate remedy, particularly at a birth when time is of the essence.

Table of Contents

Introduction to Homeopathy

Law of Similars: The Healing Principle

The word "homeopathy" means, literally, "like suffering." The idea that *a substance can cure symptoms in a sick person similar to those which it causes in a healthy person* was written about by Hypocrites, Paracelsus and Frances Bacon, and even appeared in the Hindu system of Ayurvedic medicine as far back as the tenth century B.C. The concept was rediscovered by the eighteenth century German physician Samuel Hahnemann who found that the reason quinine cured malaria was because it was capable of causing the symptoms of malaria in a healthy person. He went on to experiment with numerous natural substances, expanding the applications of this healing principle.

Law of Proving: Uncovering the Symptom Picture

All of the medicinal agents used in homeopathy have been tested or "proven" on healthy human beings. Provings involve giving repeated doses of a substance to a person and then noting any symptoms experienced. Provings can be accomplished through: (1) intentional habit, such as daily ingestion of coffee or cannabis; (2) poisoning, for example, by arsenic, mercury, bee sting or snake bite (in which cases, one "dose" is sufficient to bring out the symptom picture of the substance); or (3) a systematic process using volunteer subjects. The complete symptom picture includes changes in body tissues, physical appearance and behavior that can be observed in the person by others, as well as subjective impressions and the individual's precise description of sensations, mental attitudes and emotions.

The resulting list of symptoms, verified and updated over time by repeated provings, clinical experience and instances of poisonings, comprises the homeopathic *Materia Medica*. Numerous materia medicas have been published and continue to be published today. Typically, substances are listed in alphabetical order with detailed descriptions of their known symptom pictures. All botanicals go by their Latin, rather than common names. It is interesting to note that one criticism of herbal medicine is that we do not really know what the "side effects" of herbs are. Not true! We have 200+ years of unbiased documentation on this subject in the homeopathic materia medica. So, for example, if you are wondering whether the St. John's Wort you may be taking for depression is causing any other symptoms you may be experiencing, simply read the description of Hypericum in the homeopathic materia medica. You may just discover that you are "proving" St. John's Wort.

The homeopathic *Repertory*, on the other hand, contains a listing of substances arranged according to clinical symptoms that they are known to cause. The symptoms themselves are categorized according to body parts (such as head, back, stomach, extremities), body systems (respiratory, reproductive) and other broad categories (mind, sleep, generalities). Together with casetaking skills, the materia medica and repertory form the basis of homeopathic prescribing.

Law of Potentization: How Remedies are Made

The homeopathic pharmacopoeia today consists of over 2,000 medicines, called *remedies*. These remedies come from plant, animal and mineral sources. Hahnemann developed the pharmaceutical process for preparing homeopathic medicines. After rediscovering the Law of Similars, he endeavored to determine the *minimum dose* of a substance required to obtain a curative response, thereby reducing the occurrence of "side effects."

He began by extracting the properties of various substances. Those that were soluble in water or alcohol, he made into mother tinctures, much as herbalists do. Those that were non-soluble were triturated, or finely ground up, with powdered milk sugar as the dilutant. He then began to serially dilute the mother tincture, mixing one part tincture to nine parts dilutant. This yields a 1X potency, or a dilution of 1:10 on the decimal scale. To generate a 2X potency, he mixed one part of the 1X solution to nine parts dilutant and so on up the scale to dilutions of 200X. On the centesimal scale, the ratio is one part mother tincture to 99 parts dilutant, up to dilutions at the hundred thousandth centesimal and beyond.

Through experimentation, Hahnemann found that at some point in the dilution process, the medicines became so dilute as to have no healing effect upon the patient. Then he got the idea to *succuss*, or shake rapidly, the solution at each stage of the dilution process. The result was that the medicines became more active and stronger each time they were subjected to this process.

In a way that we do not yet fully understand, succussion releases dormant energy in matter. Hahnemann called this process *potentization*. The further removed a homeopathic remedy is from its material origin the more dynamic it becomes energetically. This dynamic, or non-material dose is thought to impart the vibrational imprint of the plant or other substance by way of the body's *vital force*. Vital force means life energy, what is *chi* to the Chinese and *prana* to the Hindus. We cannot see how the remedy works, only that it does work when the Law of Similars is skillfully applied.

In preparations beyond the 12C dilution, no molecules of the original substance can be detected in the tiny sugar pills which are the dispensing agent for the potentized tinctures. And herein lies the crux of the problem that modern science has with homeopathy: how can something so dilute as to be undetectable *by the instruments of modern physics*, nevertheless effect a medicinal action? And because they do not understand how it works and their instruments cannot measure what is happening, homeopathy is often labeled as quackery or worse by critics.

Homeopathic remedies do not saturate the bloodstream with chemical agents, but rather work on the plane of energy. Since scientists have only recently begun to find ways of measuring this energy, many orthodox practitioners attribute claims of homeopathic cures to the "placebo effect." Interestingly, one would not expect placebos to work on animals or newborn infants, but homeopathy has documented cures in both. Current research is aimed at discovering more about the energetic plane on which the remedies seem to be operating, while the efficacy of homeopathic treatment, through double-blind studies, continues to be established.

The best part of the potentization process is this: if the wrong remedy is chosen (i.e., one not based upon proper application of the Law of Similars), nothing will happen. The person's vital force will simply not respond to (or resonate with) the remedy and their symptoms will remain unaffected. So the remedies either help or they don't help, but they do no harm. Hence, they are ideal agents for use with pregnant or lactating women and infants.

An occasional (and usually short-lived) healing crisis is the worst that can happen. If such a healing crisis does result in response to a remedy, it is usually because the individual's vital force has been over stimulated. Either too high of a potency was used or the remedy was repeated too frequently. In the latter case, stop dosing. If necessary, the remedy can be antidoted (see p. 69), or you can ride out the brief aggravation. Generally, improvement will soon follow. To cause harm with homeopathy, a remedy would have to be repeated frequently as the patient's condition worsened, and then still be continued, both the prescriber and the patient demonstrating a profound lack of common sense.

It is through the process of potentization that a poison like Arsenic can be harnessed for its healing properties but pose no threat to the patient. And, indeed, the remedy Arsenicum is remarkably effective in treating food poisoning victims suffering from violent purging and diarrhea, weakness and restlessness, burning pains and anxiety—all the symptoms that Arsenic is known to cause when ingested by a healthy person in its material form.

Casetaking Hints

In order to apply the Law of Similars, the homeopathic practitioner must become a dispassionate observer of her subject. First and foremost, ***perceive the state*** the patient is in. Is she in a state of grief, anxiety, fearful apprehension, indecisiveness? Perhaps she is hypersensitive to pain, exhausted, delirious, in shock, or her hormones are in a state of imbalance. What is your main impression?

Attempt to discover the ***etiology*** of this condition. Etiologies are much broader categories in homeopathy than in standard medicine, where it is thought that most acute illnesses are caused by bacteria or viruses. In homeopathy, etiologies include emotions (such as anger, grief and fright), traumas, weather changes, foods or dietary triggers, and more. In casetaking, a clue to etiology are the words "I've never been well since ..." or similar connection of a specific stress coincident with the onset of symptoms. If the etiology is known, your choice of remedies is quickly narrowed down. For example, if all of the physical symptoms were triggered by grief, then it is the grief that needs to be treated.

What is the ***location of the problem*** and what is going on there? Is there inflammation, sepsis, spasms, discharges, retention? What is the ***sensation***? Is it burning, raw, dry, constricted, sharp pain, shooting pain? One day my four-year-old told me, "my head is cracking." He knew enough to not just say that his head hurt because that would be followed by more questions. He was trying to cut to the chase and give me a more precise description of the pain in his head.

Any factor that aggravates or ameliorates a given symptom or the person's overall condition is called a ***modality*** and is also significant. For example, pain may be made better or worse from movement, pressure, open air, or hot or cold applications. Times of day are often important modalities, many children becoming worse at night during acute illnesses. Think of the croup attack at midnight, nausea every morning, insomnia from 3–6 AM, and so on.

Any **generalities** or observations about the overall condition of the subject should also be noted. Is she pale or flushed, sweaty or dry, thirsty or not, chilly or warm, quiet or restless?

Finally, **strange, rare and peculiar symptoms** are particularly important and often provide a shortcut to the right remedy. The weirder and more precise the description of a symptom, the better the homeopath likes it. Examples include "dry mouth without thirst" or "baby ascends with contractions."

When gathering the symptom picture, refrain from over-prompting the subject and putting words in their mouth ("Is the pain a burning pain?"). Even if the answer is "yes" to this question, the symptom carries more weight if it is spontaneously reported and emphasized by the subject. Allow the reporting of symptoms to emerge, all the while using your own powers of observation. "Tell me more about the nausea and how you are feeling" is a much better opening question than "Is it worse in the morning?" For clarification purposes, you can then come around to more specific attempts to elicit information or differentiate one remedy from another.

Choosing the Remedy

Taken together, the above observations constitute the symptom picture. The cure involves matching the symptom picture of the subject to a single remedy known to cause a similar set of symptoms in a healthy person. It is important to note that it is very rare that anyone will manifest *all* the symptoms of a remedy or that all of the subject's symptoms will be mentioned in a remedy description. Your choice is based on positive matching rather than turning down a remedy because some symptoms do not match or even appear to contradict each other. In other words, if you think a remedy is a good match for the person in front of you, you should not disregard it because the materia medica lists a 9 PM aggravation time but at the moment, it is 9 AM. One mis-matched symptom does not contraindicate your remedy selection, but if the aggravation times are similar, then that is further confirmation that you may have found a good match.

Think of the stability afforded by a three-legged stool as a metaphor. Selection of a remedy based on a good match of at least three symptoms is a more stable choice than if your choice rested on one or two symptoms. These three symptoms should, at a minimum: (1) cover the main complaint and be a good match there, (2) be in the ballpark with the mental/emotional picture (e.g., Nux Vomica would be contraindicated if the person is content and sweet) and (3) match at least one modality (influences that aggravate or ameliorate the subject's symptoms).

Getting to know a remedy is like making a friend. There are certain characteristics that one notices right away. Later a few peculiarities pop up. Gradually one begins to perceive the person, to understand them and see how seemingly unrelated fragments are connected in a complex whole. The more you see them, the better you get to know them. Remedies are like that, little microcosms of the human experience. Eventually you simply recognize the remedy's personality when it is expressed in the individual before you.

Characteristics or symptoms for which a remedy are most well known are called *keynotes*. Many introductory books on homeopathy, as well as the little therapeutic manuals on specific topics (like this one), are really selective and condensed materia medicas summarizing important keynote symptoms of remedies most frequently used in clinical practice. These manuals or guides make the prescriber's job easier and are a good place to start. Someone else has narrowed down the choice. Since they are so condensed, a more extensive materia medica can be consulted if additional information is required to narrow down your selection even further (see Resources).

How Does Homeopathy Differ from Herbalism?

There is definitely some overlap in that both modalities employ botanicals. A full strength mother tincture is an herbal preparation. It is made by harvesting the plant, cleaning off any debris, placing it in a lidded jar and covering with alcohol. It is then allowed to sit for a period of six weeks to extract all its active constituents. The herbalist then filters out the plant matter and administers the resulting brown liquid by the drop or dropperful to the patient, thereby delivering a material (full strength) dose. The homeopath, however, subjects the mother tincture to the process of potentization (successive dilutions and succussion), rending it harmless but energetically activated.

The homeopath's choice of medicine always employs the Law of Similars while the herbalist may or may not be aware of the Law of Similars and may or may not be consciously applying it, even when doing so. For example, the herbalist might use tincture of Chamomile for colic or insomnia because it is known to work for these complaints. The homeopath understands that, when it works, it is because the symptoms the individual is experiencing are very close to those that Chamomile can cause when repeated doses are given to a healthy, asymptomatic person.

At the same time, it is possible for the herbalist to prescribe according to allopathic principles and most do. Allopathy literally means "opposite suffering." So, for example, allopaths give antibiotics to combat bacterial infections, anti-hypertensives to control high blood pressure, anti-depressants to overcome depression, and so on. Rather than treating the whole person, treatment is aimed at counteracting a specific problem and often different medications are targeted for different body parts or systems simultaneously. Allopathic herbalists (though none would call themselves this) also give substances that oppose symptoms.

While herbs are generally more accessible and easier to use (no poring through complex books; relatively short learning curve), homeopathy is superior because it is based on systematic employment of a proven healing principle and it is safer because it delivers an immaterial dose—energy medicine.

Midwives and Homeopathy

Like homeopaths, midwives render care to the whole person. The pregnant woman's concerns, feelings, dietary habits and physical discomforts, as well as the baby's growth, are known to be interconnected and are viewed in context. When problems surface, nourishing and gentle interventions are sought, deferring heroic measures for the rare crisis. In homeopathy, we find the perfect complement to the science and art of midwifery. It is a fascinating study. That substances exist in nature that perfectly reflect the idiosyncrasies of human beings in endless variety, and that these substances can be transformed into non-toxic medicines, is nothing short of miraculous.

Materia Medica

Aconite *(Monkshood)*

ailments brought on from a fright, such as an accident or any event capable of producing an adrenaline surge; sudden onset of symptoms; miscarriage or threatened premature birth after a fright; anxious, restless, tossings, fear of death (predicts the hour); inflammation; mom pacing in labor, afraid and needs reassurance; precipitous birth; panic state because the birth is happening fast and the midwife arrives late; sudden hemorrhage of bright blood with faintness and panic; shock state, asks "am I okay?"; shock, after the fright of a shoulder dystocia or similar emergency (give preventatively to everyone present); urine retention in the newborn or mom, especially after traumatic or precipitous delivery; sudden loss of milk supply after a fright or exposure to cold

Aethusa *(Fool's Parsley)*

#1 remedy for pyloric stenosis; projectile vomiting soon after feeding, during the early weeks of life; gas, bloating, diarrhea, weight loss, dehydration

Anacardium *(Marking Nut)*
morning sickness with dry heaves, but feels better when
eating; bowels plugged up

Antimonium Tart *(Tartrate of Antimony and Potash)*
newborn's lungs full of fluid and mucous; drowning victims; difficulty with resuscitation [use a 200C aggressively;
if responsive, continue dosing for 1–2 days, repeating only
in the case of relapse]

Apis *(Honey Bee)*
cystitis with hot stinging pains (like bee sting); scalding
pain during urination; urine retention; pruritus of pregnancy; toxemia of pregnancy with swelling; edema with
puffy face; loss of protein; high blood pressure; convulsions;
thirstlessness; better from cold applications; aggravated by
heat; jealous, irritable, mean, clumsy

Arnica *(Leopard's Bane)*
#1 first-aid remedy for trauma; bleeding, bruising, soreness,
trauma to muscles and soft tissues; helps absorb extrava-
sated blood; prevents shock; during gestation, movements
of the fetus are painful; sensation baby is lying crosswise;
varicosities with sore, aching legs, worse from pressure,
averse to stockings; bruised feeling in external genitals, extending to rectum, and aggravated by the slightest contact;
bed feels too hard; threatened miscarriage due to physical
trauma such as an accident or fall; mom doesn't want to be
touched in labor; give to mom for fetal distress occurring
when baby comes under the pubis [see also Carbo Veg];
follows any chosen hemorrhage remedy; shock state with

dazed appearance, but claims she's okay [see Aconite, "am I okay?"]; after birth, mom (or midwife!) is aching and sore all over; soreness after overexertion [see also Rhus Tox]; will help diminish afterpains [see also Mag Phos]; urine retention due to swelling; speeds healing of the perineum; give as soon as possible to breech or premature babies; give to any baby upset after difficult birth; will heal hematoma quickly; actually, just give to all moms and babies after delivery [should be continued until any soreness, bruising, or swelling is completely resolved]

Arsenicum *(Iodide of Arsenic)*

chilly, anxious, fearful, restless; insomnia, aggravation between midnight and 3 AM; morning sickness; heartburn at pylorus; thirsty but can't drink much, food smells terrible; severe vomiting and diarrhea due to food poisoning, even to bringing on miscarriage or premature labor; rigidity of vagina, will hardly admit a finger; mother cleans house fanatically in labor; exhaustion, prostration; lack of progress in labor in fearful, fastidious, compulsive women who can't let go; newborn resuscitation in severely depressed baby with little or no color or respiratory effort [see Moskowitz book for case studies]

Belladonna *(Deadly Nightshade)*

fever with hot, red face; glassy eyes with dilated pupils; bounding pulse; bursting headache; twitching; moaning; delirious; wants to escape (freaking out); worse from light, motion, jarring the bed, noise; extremely sensitive to touch; symptoms come on suddenly; hot, moist, thin, rigid cervix; back labor, feels as though it would break; phlebitis with

red, hot, swollen and throbbing veins; forceful, gushing
hemorrhage with hot, bright red bleeding, spasms, and
great sensitivity; blood feels hot; fever relieved during
hemorrhage; violent convulsions, head to toe, during or
after delivery; milk fever, copious flow of milk; mastitis
with fever and red areas or streaks on the breast; breasts very
tender and swollen, with throbbing pain [Phytolacca often
follows Belladonna in breast infections, after the fever stage]

Bellis Perennis *(Daisy)*
inability to walk during pregnancy; pain down anterior of
thighs; uterus sore, uncomfortable, as if squeezed; soreness
of abdominal wall during pregnancy; bearing down sensation, feels as if she must hold her belly up [also Sepia];
varicosities; dragging afterpains; often in multips with weak
abdominal muscles; prolapsed rectum; similar to Arnica for
bruises, contusion, hematoma, called "Arnica of the abdo-
men"; [follows Staphysagria and Arnica after cesarean, for
pains and to speed recovery; see pp. 55–56]

Borax *(Borate of Sodium)*
thrush; baby's mouth sore, cries when nursing or refuses
to nurse; dread of descending or downward motion (baby
cries and clings to mom when being placed in crib or on
forward motion of baby swing, etc.); apthae on nipples of
nursing mom

Bryonia *(Wild Hops)*
phlebitis with red, hot, swollen veins and aching pain,
better from pressure and tight wrapping, but worse any
motion; engorged breasts, will reduce excessive milk at

onset; painful breast infections with fever; breast stony hard with sharp, stitching pains; all symptoms worse from movement; mom holds breast when going up or down stairs; very irritable, wants to be alone, averse to stimulation; very thirsty with dry mucous membranes; symptoms come on slowly [Phytolacca often follows in breast infections, after the fever]

Calcarea Carbonica *(Carbonate of Lime)*
shortness of breath, worse climbing stairs; pica—craves dirt, chalk, coal, pencils and other indigestibles; irresistible desire to smell carbon-based products (such as magic markers, gasoline, etc.); likes eggs and dairy products; constipated, but usually not uncomfortable with it; varicosities of the vulva; varices of the bladder causing blood in the urine; chilly; sweats easily, especially head, chest and feet; responsible and task-oriented; insomnia due to worry; milk supply regulator; restores milk supply after an acute illness; #1 for umbilical hernia; big children's remedy—chronic colic, thrush, yeast diaper rash, developmental delays, difficult or late teething, chronic snuffles due to milk allergy, constipation, stork bites, spina bifida, cradle cap [see Paul Herscu's book, *The Homeopathic Treatment of Children* for a good description of the infant type]

Calcarea Fluorica *(Fluoride of Lime)*
See Tissues Salts (p. 36)

Calcarea Phosphorica *(Phosphate of Lime)*
See Tissue Salts (p. 36)

Calendula *(Marigold)*

often used as an external application; diluted mother tincture (1/10) stops bleeding when applied to cervical or vaginal tears; one dropperful of mother tincture in full peri bottle applied to torn perineum or incision site 3–5 times per day speeds healing and prevents infection; water infusion of the flower tops added to postpartum bath heals tears quickly; can be used in oil base on stitches to prevent irritation from the pad; in cream or oil base for sore nipples; various preparations also helpful for umbilical stumps that are slow to heal or showing signs of infection; topically for diaper rash; give in potency in cases of poor wound healing

Cantharis *(Spanish Fly)*

#1 remedy for cystitis; fever, urging, and frequency with urination; bloody urine; burning or cutting pains; dribbling after urination; burning of labia, worse after urination; retained placenta with painful urination

Carbo Vegetabilis *(Vegetable Charcoal)*

sluggishness and indigestion with bloating; much gas with belching and flatus; shortness of breath, worse flatus and overeating, better belching; varicosities of the leg, thigh, vulva; edema and stasis ulcers, cold to touch; phlebitis; hemorrhage with paleness and icy coldness of body; fainting; air hunger, yawning, wants to be fanned; weak, sluggish, exhausted, lack of stamina; to improve oxygenation of newborn; give during labor for decelerations in FHT; collapsed, limp, flaccid, cold, appears dead; known as homeopathic "corpse reviver"

Castor Equi *(Rudimentary Thumbnail of the Horse)*
#1 remedy for cracked and ulcerated nipples; deep, painful
cracks, excessively tender; areola reddened; violent itching
in breasts

Caulophyllum *(Blue Cohosh)*
first trimester miscarriages due to uterine weakness from
repeated abortions, miscarriages and childbirths; excessive
toning contractions prior to labor; known as a labor regulator [alternate with Cimicifuga; also with mother tinctures
of each]; to initiate or augment contractions; painful,
spasmodic contractions, with shivering or inner trembling
and lack of progress; irregular, strong, but ineffective contractions on a rigid cervix; contractions feel like pinpricks;
pains flag from exhaustion; tremulous weakness, prostration; nervous and nauseous with stomach spasms; hemorrhage and/or retained placenta due to absent contractions
or uterine weakness, usually after long labor; uterus soft and
flabby; painful, swollen joints of the fingers or toes during
pregnancy or postpartum; may diminish afterpains

Causticum *(Hahnemann's Tinctura acris sine Kali)*
urinary stress incontinence; burning, rawness, and soreness;
uterine inertia during labor; contractions insufficient and
irregular; distressing back pain in labor; long, slow labor
with over-stretched bladder; retention from long holding
of the urine or after catheterization; great sympathy for
the suffering of others; idealistic, political women who are
incensed over injustices

Chamomilla *(German Chamomile)*

hypersensitivity to pain, cannot bear it; coffee withdrawal headaches; restless, impatient, cross, ugly, spiteful, snappish; capricious, wants attention but nothing satisfies; angry with attendants; bites attendants; whiny, throws partner out of the room; thirsty; labor pains unendurable yet unproductive, shooting upwards; rigid cervical os; constant tearing pains in back, not just with contractions; excellent remedy for newborns and infants; jaundice with irritability; acute colic episodes with arching of back, kicking and screaming; baby refuses to nurse, screams instead; teething problems with fever and fretfulness; one cheek red/hot, the other pale/cold; inconsolable infants want to be carried; worse 9 PM; restless sleep, wakes often

Chelidonium *(Celandine)*

during pregnancy, pain underneath right scapula; gallbladder pain; long-lasting jaundice in newborn; baby sleepy, not nursing well, soft muscle tone

Cimicifuga *(Black Cohosh)*

helps produce coordinated contractions [alternate with Caulophyllum; also with mother tinctures of each]; cervix dilated then closed; shivers during first stage of labor; lack of progress in labor with displaced labor pains; pains fly from side to side, across the pelvis; cramps in hips, shooting pains into thighs; sciatica; twitching and trembling of legs; overly sensitive, cannot tolerate pain; foreboding that something bad is going to happen, especially in women who have had previous traumatic birth experiences; loquacious and hysterical; great anxiety, fear of going insane

Cinchona *(Peruvian Bark—China)*
reviver; faintness after loss of body fluids (bleeding, diarrhea, vomiting); loss of sight, ringing in ears; cold sweat with weakness and pallor; aversion to being touched; mother still feels dragged out after day three or is weak from long labor

Cocculus *(Indian Cockle)*
nausea aggravated by riding in cars, as in motion sickness; vertigo accompanies nausea; sensitive to smell or thought of food; insomnia from night watching and caring for others

Coffea *(Unroasted Coffee)*
hypersensitive to noise or vibration; nervous, fearful; insomnia due to excitement, racing thoughts, activity of the mind; slightest noise awakens; great sensitivity; agonizing labor pains with sciatica; back labor; decreased milk due to excitement

Colchicum *(Meadow Saffron)*
nausea of pregnancy; great sensitivity to odors; aversion to meat, eggs and fish; thought of food is gross; abdominal distension with trapped gas; retching and vomiting; diarrhea; toxemia, protein in the urine, edema

Colocynthis *(Bitter Cucumber)*
acute colic episodes; tries to bend forward or pulls legs up to belly; better from hard pressure and warmth; better lying face downwards; moaning between spasms

Ferrum Phosphoricum *(Phosphate of Iron)*
See Tissue Salts (p. 36)

Gelsemium *(Yellow Jasmine)*

post-dates anxiety especially in primips; complaints from anticipation of an event; performance anxiety; on-again/off-again labor; thick, rigid cervix; great fatigue and weakness; nervous chattering; spasmodic pains; dilation at a standstill; pains move up and down the back; trembling, especially legs, from the slightest exertion; dull, dazed, weak; mom drops things; absent urge to push, baby ascends with contractions; incoordinate muscular action; retained urine after delivery; performance anxiety in midwives (nervousness, shaking, frequent stools)

Gossypium *(Cotton Plant)*

sluggish second stage of labor; retained placenta, especially after miscarriage or premature delivery with closed os

Graphites *(Black Lead)*

nipples sore, cracked and blistered [if Castor Equi fails]; eruptions in axilla, under breasts; especially in obese women; may aid in reabsorption of scar tissue [see also Silica and Thiosinaminum]

Hamamelis *(Witch Hazel)*

#1 remedy for varicose veins and hemorrhoids; lax ligaments and tissues; bruising and ecchymosis [also Arnica]; veins are sore and irritated with stinging pain; congested, hard and knotty, swollen, heavy; sensitive to touch; varicosities of the vulva; bleeding hemorrhoids [use in potency and locally as an ointment or compress with tincture]; phlebitis; passive hemorrhage due to weak veins; prolapsed rectum

Hepar Sulph *(Calcium Sulphide)*
vaginitis; discharge is curdy and smells sour or like old cheese, with itching and great irritation of tissues; mastitis with pus production; conjunctivitis in the newborn [if Pulsatilla fails] with yellow-green discharge and redness of upper eyelid; great sensitivity to cold; better from warmth; irritable and hypersensitive to pain and touch

Hydrastis *(Goldenseal)*
sinusitis or vaginitis; thick, yellow, ropy discharge; itchy vulva; intercourse relieves

Hypericum *(St. John's Wort)*
#1 first-aid remedy for trauma to nerves; radiating pain from sight of injury; convulsions from trauma to the head or spine; give to baby prophylactically after dystocia or traumatic delivery [see also Arnica]; for pain after cesarean delivery [see pp. 55–56]; pain in tailbone since childbirth, or broken tailbone

Ignatia *(St. Ignatius Bean)*
for acute grief states with weeping and much sighing; idealistic, romantic, or hysterical women; emotions become "unhinged" after prolonged stress; miscarriage due to grief; sleepless from grief; loss of appetite; feeling of a lump in the throat or a sore throat after a disappointment; twitching and spasms in labor; grimacing; postpartum depression, especially in women who may have had an overly romanticized notion of birth and were shocked by the reality; when birth outcomes fall short of the mom's ideal [see also Staphysagria if feeling victimized]; decreased milk due to emotional upset

Ipecac *(Ipecac Root)*
    morning sickness with clean tongue and excess salivation;
    incapacitating nausea with retching; nausea unrelieved by
    vomiting; hyperemesis; averse to all food; stomach seems to
    hang loose inside; ptyalism in pregnancy [see also Pulsa-
    tilla]; threatened miscarriage due to extreme nausea and
    vomiting [see also Arsenicum]; repeated vomiting in labor;
    hemorrhage with nausea and vomiting; bright red, profuse
    uterine bleeding, comes in gushes

Kali Bichromicum *(Bichromate of Potash)*
    sinusitis or vaginitis with yellow-green, thick, gluey, stringy
    discharge; itching and burning of vulva; left-sided sciatica;
    chronic snuffles of fat, chubby babies

Kali Carbonicum *(Carbonate of Potassium)*
    severe backache during pregnancy or accompanying
    miscarriage; right-sided sciatica; sleep disturbed by back
    pain; back labor radiating to gluteal muscles and legs, better
    pressure; swelling over eyes; depressed and irritable postpar-
    tum, with back pain; worse change in weather

Kali Phosphoricum *(Phosphate of Potash)*
    See Tissue Salts (p. 37)

Kreosotum *(Beechwood Kreosote)*
    vaginitis with burning, excoriating discharge; foul odor;
    persistent, violent itching of the vulva and vagina, can
    extend to thighs; vulva burns when urine passes

Lac Caninum *(Dog's Milk)*
    to dry up milk [try 30C potency for several days; wean off

remedy gradually to prevent rebound lactation effect; see also Pulsatilla]; vertigo, floating sensation; mastitis that travels from left breast to right breast and back to the left; symptoms alternate sides of the body

Lac Defloratum *(Skimmed Milk)*
migraine headaches, worse during pregnancy; migraine with visual aura; one-sided throbbing frontal headache; sick headache; nausea of pregnancy with motion sickness and constipation

Lactuca Virosa *(Acrid Lettuce)*
deficient or absent milk; a true galactagogue; for women adopting a baby who want to nurse [consult a lactation consultant as well]; to increase milk supply or relactate [try frequent doses of 30C or lower potency]

Laurocerasus *(Cherry Laurel)*
infant resuscitation; face blue; difficulty breathing, gasping for breath; pulse failing; heart abnormalities

Lycopodium *(Club Moss)*
low self-esteem or lack of self-confidence, anxious; kidney pain, worse on right or starts on right and moves to the left; huge appetite with bloating and distension; trapped intestinal gas, with sharp pains; heartburn; painful varicosities of the leg, thigh, vulva; newborn complaints include chronic colic, chronic obstruction of nasal passages, wild nursers with hiccoughs, jaundice, birth anomalies in the urogenital tract, undescended testicles, right-sided hernias [see Paul Herscu's book, *The Homeopathic Treatment of Children* for a

good description of the infant type; also recommendations
for hernias in the newborn]

Magnesia Phosphorica *(Phosphate of Magnesia)*
See Tissue Salts (p. 37)

Medorrhinum *(Gonorrhea Nosode)*
chronic sinusitis, vaginitis or cystitis; may date back to
beginning a new sexual relationship; in women who have
a history of pot smoking, numerous sexual partners or
sexually transmitted disease, especially gonorrhea; vaginal
discharge thin, acrid, excoriating, fishy odor [also Sanicula];
intense pruritus of the genitals; warts on genitals; herpes;
infertility and a history of STD; mentally spacey, difficult
concentration; loves stimulation, loud music and partying;
chronic and sharply demarcated diaper rash in babies; babies sleep in the knee-chest position, with butt up in the air

Natrum Muriaticum *(Chloride of Sodium)*
infertility due to long-standing grief; excessive dryness or
moisture in any part of system; too little or too much amniotic fluid; can help turn a breech, transverse or posterior
baby if position is due to too little or too much fluid [see p.
53]; craves salt; coldness of body, especially legs and feet;
heartburn; constipation; vaginitis, discharge watery and
like egg white; #1 remedy for herpes; herpes brought on by
emotional stress and fatigue; deep depression, fear of rejection; history of being disappointed in relationships; mom
emotionally blocked up with grief and worry; emotions
walled off, stoic behavior; behind her wall, mom feels very

vulnerable; consolation aggravates, wants to be alone to cry or suddenly bursts into tears after much suppression

Natrum Phosphoricum *(Phosphate of Sodium)*
See Tissue Salts (p. 37)

Natrum Sulphuricum *(Sulphate of Sodium)*
history of head injury; nausea; gas, bloating, desires sweets; headache with constipation; yellow vaginal discharge; tissue salt (in 6X potency) which governs liver function and regulates the amount of water in the tissues; will help eliminate excess water; woman feels overburdened and overwhelmed, life is a struggle; postpartum depression; jaundice in the newborn; worse hot, humid weather

Nitricum Acidum *(Nitric Acid)*
over-indulgence in sugar; also craves chalk, earth and other indigestibles; loves fat and salt; canker sores; irritable

Nux Vomica *(Poison Nut)*
morning sickness; feels like a hangover; toxic feeling with nausea and vomiting; dry heaves, retching; hypersensitive to noise and odors; very chilly; ineffectual urging described as "wants to (pass stool, vomit, urinate, be delivered) but can't"; constipated, sluggish; dull, toxic headache; insomnia, can't turn mind off, worse after 3 AM; irritability with backache and spasms; impatient, fault-finding, abusive, nasty; lots of stress in overworked, hard-driving women; irritable, sensitive babies with constipation and straining, better after a bowel movement

Opium *(Dried Latex of the Poppy)*
resuscitation; respiration slow, noisy, obstructed; Cheyne-Stokes respiration; makes a puffing sound with each respiration; heavy, stuporous appearance; face flushed deep red or mottled purple; eyes heavy and half closed, pupils constricted, staring; jaw drooping; sweaty skin; twitching limbs; constipation or urine retention in the newborn; aggravation from a fright; bad effects from anesthesia

Phosphorus
bleeding gums or nosebleeds during pregnancy; diabetes; hyperemesis of pregnancy [see also Ipecac]; vomiting in labor, as soon as food or drink warms up in the stomach; post-surgical vomiting due to effects of anesthesia [see pp. 55–56]; profuse hemorrhage in tall, slim, fine-featured women; bright-red bleeding with intense thirst; craves ice cold drinks, sweets, ice cream; sparkling, extroverted and sympathetic women who want company; anxious when alone

Phytolacca *(Poke Root)*
#1 remedy for breast infections [often follows Belladonna or Bryonia after the fever stage]; nipples sore and fissured; intense suffering on putting child to breast; pain radiates all over body; breast feels like a brick, lumpy and nodular, caked, blocked ducts; excessive milk flow; mammary abscess [see also Silica]; irritable, restless, indifferent, sure she will die; backache and fever, chilly and shivering; recurrent mastitis [use high potency]

Pulsatilla *(Wind Flower)*
weepy and emotional, cries readily; mild symptoms;

indecisive, impressionable, contradictory, changeable;
wants/demands constant attention and reassurance; aggravation in a hot, stuffy room; better fresh air and gentle
movement; nausea later in the day, usually in response
to fatty foods, which she craves; nausea accompanied by
persistent headaches during pregnancy; better cold foods;
dry mouth but thirstless; ptyalism [see also Ipecac]; vaginitis, changeable discharge, usually creamy with burning;
varicosities of the leg, thigh, foot, with stinging pains; limbs
lain on become numb and cold; phlebitis; threatening
miscarriage with changeable symptoms; to aid a miscarriage
to completion, often with bleeding that stops and starts,
or with retained placenta; may help change a posterior or
breech presentation [see pp. 53–54]; weak, ineffective,
irregular contractions appear suddenly and gradually dis-
appear; pains erratic, accompanied by shivering and tears;
lack of progress in labor; simultaneous heat and coldness in
parts of body; woman calls out for her mommy in labor;
retained placenta; postpartum hemorrhage starts and stops
repeatedly, usually beginning again when the midwife
diverts her attention from the mom; postpartum weepiness;
may help regulate overabundant supply or aberrant milk
production; overactive letdown reflex; cracked nipples with
pain extending down back or pain changes from place to
place; breastmilk in the newborn; #1 remedy for newborn
conjunctivitis [see also Hepar Sulph]

Pyrogenium *(Artificial Sepsin)*
uterine infection; sepsis; low fever with rapid pulse or high
fever with slow pulse; restless; chill begins in the back;

profuse hot sweat; dark, offensive blood; throbbing headache; whole body aches, bed feels too hard; better warmth

Rhus Tox *(Poison Ivy)*
insomnia with tossing and turning, worse around midnight; restless, can't get comfortable; back and joints ache;
sciatica; restless legs at night; stiff in the morning but better
once one is up and moving about; fingers swollen and stiff
in the morning; pruritus; ailments brought on by overexertion [also Arnica], especially in the cold and damp; stiffness
predominates; threatened miscarriage after exposure or
overexertion; strained and chilled after long labor; better
from hot baths, warmth in any form, massage, movement;
midwife stiff and achy after overexertion at a birth; cures
shingles [amazing! had to add this, though admittedly not a
pregnancy/birth-related ailment]

Ricinus *(Castor Oil)*
increases the quantity of milk in nursing women; languor
and weakness [Boericke recommends low potencies repeated every 4 hours; also locally a poultice of the leaves]

Ruta Graveolens *(Rue Bitterwort)*
miscarriages at seven months; stiffness in muscles and ten-
dons, especially after injury; prolapsed rectum after delivery

Sabina *(Savine)*
#1 to assist miscarriage with bright red bleeding mixed with
clots; worse from least motion; also used to treat chronic
tendency to miscarriage in the third month; pain radiates
from sacrum or low back to the pubis; retained placenta;

uterine atony; desires fresh air, lemonade; endometriosis source of uterine problems

Sambucus *(Elder)*
nasal obstruction; snuffles in newborns preventing nursing; cold feet with warm body; perspires over whole body, but not the head; better when upright; better motion

Sanicula *(Aqua)*
vaginitis with odor of fish-brine or old cheese [see also Hepar Sulph]

Sarsaparilla *(Smilax)*
cystitis with pain at the end of urination; burning and frequency; nipples small, withered, retracted or inverted

Secale *(Ergot)*
prolonged bearing down pains without results; hemorrhage; passive flow of dark, thin blood from low-lying placenta; to clamp down lower segment of uterus; tremendous burning and heat; better from cold and uncovering, though skin feels cold to the touch; often thin, feeble multips

Sepia *(Inky Juice of Cuttlefish)*
infertility or periodic miscarriages due to hormonal imbalances; never well since taking the birth control pill; never well since any big hormonal change (e.g., puberty, pregnancy, weaning, menopause); mask of pregnancy; irritable, dragged-out fatigue; dutiful women with flat or ambivalent emotions; aversion to and irritability with family members; wants to be left alone; worse from housework, sex, demands of the children; better vigorous exercise, loves to

dance; chilly; insatiable hunger, then nauseous; worse from smell of food; constipation with a sense of weight or ball in rectum; persistent sinus problems or cough during pregnancy; varicosities; vaginitis with greenish-yellow discharge; intercourse is extremely painful; herpes; poor muscle tone with uterine prolapse, incompetent cervix, placenta previa, urinary incontinence; bearing down sensation in the pelvis as if everything will just fall out; uterus sore from activity of fetus; weakness in small of back, achy, tired feeling, better pressure; postpartum depression with aversion to or rejection of baby; deep, sore cracks across crown of nipple

Silica *(Pure Flint)*
See Tissue Salts (pp. 37–38)

Staphysagria *(Stavesacre)*
obstructed labor in abused women with suppressed anger, indignation; history of rape, victimization or other abuse; mom doesn't want to be touched in labor [see also Arnica]; trauma of cut or torn tissues (episiotomies, bad tears, cesareans); stretched sphincter pain after catheterization; will help expel incarcerated gas after cesarean delivery; relieves pain in the incision site (even weeks or months later) [see pp. 55–56]; oversensitive, angry, brooding, silent martyr; tries to please; postpartum depression in moms with unexpressed anger, perhaps after experiencing birth as a form of abuse; nursing almost impossible from pain when milk begins to flow; colic in baby due to mother's suppressed anger [treat the mother]

Sulphur *(Sublimated Sulphur)*
  generally warm and aggravated by heat; skin eruptions of all
  kinds, with itching and burning, worse after a bath; diarrhea; catnap sleep, wakes frequently from itching or heat;
  toxemia of late pregnancy with edema, hypertension

Symphoricarpus *(Snowberry)*
  persistent vomiting of pregnancy; nausea, water brash, bitter taste, averse to all food; constipation; worse any motion;
  better lying on back

Thiosinaminum *(A Chemical Derived from Oil of
Mustard Seed)*
  dissolves scar tissue [see also Graphites and Silica];
  abdominal adhesions arising from endometriosis, PID,
  abdominal surgery

Tuberculinum *(from Tubercular Abscess)*
  birth defects point to the need for this remedy; especially
  defects of the midline, the spine or palate; baby born with
  teeth, or child has extra or missing teeth; tongue-tied; babies are born with dark or long, fine hair on scalp and along
  the spine and long eyelashes [see Paul Herscu's book, *The
  Homeopathic Treatment of Children*, for a good description
  of the infant type]

Urtica Urens *(Stinging Nettle)*
  absent, deficient, or inappropriate lactation; skin eruptions with sensitivity and burning, stinging, itching pains;
  pruritus vulva

Tissue Salts

THE TWELVE HOMEOPATHIC TISSUE SALTS (also known as biochemics or cell salts) are the inorganic constituents of body tissues and fluids. According to Dr. Schuessler's theory of biochemistry, the ability of the body cells to assimilate, excrete and utilize nutrients from food is impaired if there is a deficiency in the inorganic mineral constituent of the cellular tissues. Normal cell metabolism can be restored by supplying the required tissue salts in their finely divided, easily assimilated form.

The tissue salts work, therefore, on a nutritional level within the body and are a subset of homeopathic remedies. They can be used safely over a longer period of time and with greater frequency than one would normally take a homeopathic remedy. Typically they are taken 2–3 times per day for a period of 1–4 weeks, depending upon the severity of the deficiency. Often it can be helpful to use two tissue salts at once. In this case, each remedy is taken twice daily, in alternation.

Tissue salts are usually given in a 6X potency, though they are also sold in 3X and 12X. When used in higher potencies the remedy is no longer considered to be a tissue salt. *The*

Biochemic Handbook by Formur, Inc. is an inexpensive resource book containing more information on use of the tissue salts.

Following is a brief symptom picture of the tissue salts most frequently indicated in midwifery practice. Both Natrum Muriaticum and Natrum Sulphuricum are also tissue salts. I have not included them in this section because I more often use them in higher potency.

Calcarea Fluorica *(Fluoride of Lime)*
governs elasticity of tissues and walls of blood vessels; relaxed condition of elastic fibers; useful in varicose veins and hemorrhoids; stretch marks; large and hard uterine fibroids; may prevent formation of adhesions after cesarean [see pp. 55–56]

Calcarea Phosphorica *(Phosphate of Lime)*
general nutrient; impaired digestion, mal-assimilation; improves absorption of calcium; eliminates tendency for leg cramps [alternate with Mag Phos]; pain in the symphysis pubis during pregnancy; increases milk supply; mother run down from prolonged nursing; teething problems; delayed development; failure to thrive in babies; infant wants to nurse all of the time and vomits easily; child refuses breast, milk tastes salty

Ferrum Phosphoricum *(Phosphate of Iron)*
oxygen carrier; anemia; improves absorption of iron; builds hemoglobin after hemorrhage [give 3 doses daily for a week or more along with iron-rich foods and herbs]

Kali Phosphoricum *(Phosphate of Potash)*
nerve nutrient; exhaustion in labor [try frequent doses, between contractions, for an hour or so]; may also be helpful for nervous exhaustion in the postpartum period

Magnesia Phosphorica *(Phosphate of Magnesia)*
nerve stabilizer; main remedy for nervous complaints of a spasmodic nature; ailments characterized by intense, darting, spasmodic, cramping pains [use in alternation with Calc Phos for various cramping complaints during pregnancy]; leg cramps in labor; for afterpains, put two tablets in a cup of hot water and have mom sip on it as needed, especially when the baby is nursing; acute colic pains with flatulence; doubling up with pain; pains are better from heat, warm drinks, pressure

Natrum Phosphoricum *(Phosphate of Sodium)*
acid neutralizer; ailments that arise from an acid condition of the system; after too much sugar; indigestion, heartburn, sour vomiting; tongue has thick yellow coating; rheumatic pain

Silica *(Pure Flint)*
cleanser; stimulates the absorption of scar tissue [see also Graphites and Thiosinaminum]; sore nipples, cracked, ulcerated, don't heal; #1 for breast abscesses, baby rejects milk on that side [go to a higher potency if the tissue salt doesn't clear symptoms]; plugged tear ducts in newborn; delayed development; failure to thrive, especially in premature infants who cannot assimilate nutrients; frequent vomiting of breastmilk with weight loss; infected umbilicus with

pus production; chilly and weak; ***one warning with this remedy*** *is that it can expel foreign objects in the body, hence its effective use in a case of an embedded splinter, but should not be used with folks who have surgically implanted pins, tubes and so on*

Repertory

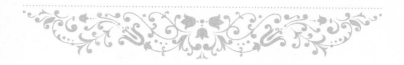

Remedies Listed According to Therapeutic Applications

* indicates that the remedy is a leading remedy for the problem listed

PRENATAL PROBLEMS

❧ **Anemia**
　Ferrum Phos

❧ **Bleeding Gums/ Nosebleeds**
　Phosphorus

❧ **Chloasma** *(mask of pregnancy)*
　Sepia

❧ **Constipation**
　Anacardium
　Calc Carb
　Lac Defloratum
　Natrum Mur
　Natrum Sulph
　Nux Vomica*
　Sepia*
　Symphoricarpus

❧ **Discomforts**

　　back pain
　　　Kali Carb
　　　Nux Vomica
　　　Sepia

　　bearing down or funneling sensation in pelvis
　　　Bellis
　　　Sepia*

excessive toning contractions
Calc Phos
Caulophyllum
Mag Phos

gallbladder pain
Chelidonium

joints stiff
Rhus tox

leg cramps
Calc Phos
Mag Phos

movements of fetus painful
Arnica
Sepia

restless legs
Rhux Tox

sciatica
Cimicifuga
Coffea
Kali Bich
Kali Carb
Rhus Tox

symphysis pubis, pain
Calc Phos

uterus sore
Arnica
Bellis

❧ **Dyspnea** *(shortness of breath)*
Calc Carb
Carbo Veg

❧ **Headaches**
Belladonna
Chamomilla
Lac Defloratum
Natrum Sulph
Nux Vomica
Pulsatilla

❧ **Herpes**
Medorrhinum
Natrum Mur*
Sepia

❧ **Infertility** *(see also Miscarriage/Chronic Tendency)*
Medorrhinum
Natrum Mur
Sepia

❧ **Insomnia**
Arsenicum
Calc Carb
Chamomilla
Cocculus
Coffea*
Ignatia
Kali Carb

Nux Vomica*
Rhus Tox*
Sulphur

❧ **Mal-Presentation of the Baby** *(see also pp. 53–54)*
Natrum Mur
Pulsatilla*

❧ **Morning Sickness/ Indigestion**
Anacardium
Arsenicum
Carbo Veg
Cocculus*
Colchicum
Kali Mur
Lac Defloratum
Lycopodium
Natrum Sulph
Nux Vomica*
Pulsatilla*
Sepia*
Symphoricarpus

food poisoning
Arsenicum

heartburn
Arsenicum
Lycopodium
Natrum Mur
Natrum Phos

hyperemesis
Ipecac*
Phosphorus

❧ **Phlebitis**
Belladonna
Bryonia
Carbo Veg
Hamamelis
Pulsatilla

❧ **Pica** *(craving for non-food substances)*
Calc Carb*
Nitric Acid

❧ **Pruritus**
Apis
Rhus Tox
Sulphur
Urtica Urens

❧ **Ptyalism** *(excess salivation)*
Ipecac
Pulsatilla*

❧ **Scar Tissue/Stretch Marks**

prevention
Calc Fluor

reabsorption
Graphites
Silica
Thiosinaminum

❧ Sinusitis
Hydrastis
Kali Bich*
Medorrhinum
Sepia*

❧ Sugar in the Urine
Phosphorus
Pulsatilla

❧ Toxemia
Apis
Colchicum
Nux Vomica
Sulphur

❧ Urinary Tract Infections
Apis
Cantharis*
Causticum
Lycopodium
Medorrhinum
Sarsaparilla

❧ Vaginitis
Hepar Sulph
Hydrastis
Kali Bich
Kreosotum*
Medorrhinum
Natrum Mur
Natrum Sulph
Pulsatilla*

Sanicula
Sepia*

❧ Varicose Veins
Arnica
Bellis
Calc Fluor*
Carbo Veg
Hamamelis*
Lycopodium
Pulsatilla*
Sepia*

of the bladder
Calc Carb

of the vulva
Calc Carb
Carbo Veg
Hamamelis
Lycopodium

POSTPARTUM/MOM

❧ **Afterpains**
Arnica
Bellis
Caulophyllum
Mag Phos*

❧ **Depression/Emotions**
Ignatia
Kali Carb
Kali Phos
Natrum Mur
Natrum Sulph
Pulsatilla*
Sepia*
Staphysagria

❧ **Phlebitis**
Belladonna
Bryonia
Carbo Veg
Hamamelis
Pulsatilla

❧ **Prolapsed Rectum**
Hamamelis
Ruta
Sepia

❧ **Prolapsed Uterus**
Sepia

❧ **Scar Tissue**
prevention
Calc Fluor
reabsorption
Graphites
Silica
Thiosinaminum

❧ **Uterine Infection/ Sepsis**
Belladonna
Pyrogenium

❧ **Urinary Stress Incontinence**
Causticum
Sepia*

POSTPARTUM/BABY

❧ **Birth Defects**
Calc Carb
Laurocerasus
Lycopodium
Tuberculinum

❧ **Breastmilk in the Newborn**
Pulsatilla

❧ **Colic**
Chamomilla*
Colocynthis*
Mag Phos*
Staphysagria

chronic
Calc Carb*
Lycopodium*

❧ **Constipation**
Calc Carb
Nux Vomica*
Opium

❧ **Cradle Cap**
Calc Carb

❧ **Developmental Delays**
Calc Carb
Calc Phos
Silica

❧ **Diaper Rash**
Calc Carb
Calendula
Medorrhinum

❧ **Eyes**
blocked tear ducts
Silica

conjunctivitis
Hepar Sulph
Pulsatilla*

❧ **Failure to Thrive**
Calc Phos
Silica

❧ **Hernia**
Calc Carb

❧ **Jaundice**
Chamomilla
Chelidonium
Lycopodium
Natrum Sulph

❧ **Nasal Congestion**
Calc Carb
Kali Bich
Lycopodium
Sambucus

❧ Pyloric Stenosis
Aethusa

❧ Teething
Calc Carb
Calc Phos
Chamomilla

❧ Thrush
Borax
Calc Carb

BREASTFEEDING

❧ Engorgement
Bryonia

❧ Mastitis
Belladonna*
Bryonia*
Lac Caninum
Phytolacca*

abscesses in breast
Hepar Sulph
Silica*

❧ Milk Supply Decreased or Absent
Aconite
Calc Carb
Calc Phos
Coffea
Ignatia
Lactuca Virosa*
Pulsatilla
Ricinus
Urtica Urens

❧ Sore Nipples/Painful Nursing
Borax
Calendula*
Castor Equi*
Graphites
Phytolacca
Pulsatilla
Sepia
Silica
Staphysagria

❧ To Dry Up Milk Supply
Lac Caninum*
Pulsatilla

Homeopathic Preparation for Delivery

Pre-eminent Female Remedies

Natrum Muriaticum, Pulsatilla and Sepia are the three most commonly seen female remedies. Many women will change to a Pulsatilla type when pregnant. Midwives may enjoy familiarizing themselves with these remedies by reading about them in depth. See Richard Moskowitz's *Homeopathic Medicines for Pregnancy and Childbirth* and Catherine Coulter's *Portraits of Homeopathic Medicines*. If women are presenting a strong picture of a remedy during pregnancy, difficulties during labor and birth may be averted with prenatal treatment in high potency. For example, the Pulsatilla hemorrhage or Sepia's uterine prolapse may not occur if the midwife learns to recognize and treat the less dramatic symptoms prenatally. If prophylaxis works, we can only know that we have done no harm. Dramatic evidence of positive response eludes us as we practice the art of prevention. It is only in hindsight, after the more serious complication occurs, that we can sometimes perceive the full symptom picture that was present all along.

Recommended Prenatal Regimen

Many homeopaths recommend that the following remedies be taken during the last month of pregnancy to help prepare the woman for labor. Not all women require that preventive measures be taken, but there are some who will benefit. I particularly encourage all of my first-time mothers and women who have a history of post-dates pregnancies, dysfunctional labors with failure to progress or unusually long labors to undertake this regimen. The woman should start taking the remedies four weeks prior to her due date. She takes each remedy once per week, alternating as follows: Caulophyllum on Monday, Cimicifuga on Wednesday, and Arnica on Friday.

Caulophyllum 12C or 30C (whatever you have on hand)
  natural source of oxytocin; helps produce effective contractions; can be used to initiate or enhance labor; will not bring on contractions if the woman is not ready to go into labor and may relieve excessive pre-labor toning contractions

Cimicifuga 12C or 30C
  to ease fear of giving birth; complements the action of Caulophyllum by aiding the uterus to contract in a coordinated and effective way; especially helpful for women with past traumatic birth experiences who have a sense of impending doom about the approaching labor

Arnica 12C or 30C
  to avoid the physical trauma associated with childbirth; prevents excess blood loss, shock and trauma to soft tissues; often used prophylactically prior to surgery, dental treatments and so on

To Change an Unfavorable Presentation Prior to Onset of Labor

Approximately four weeks before the due date, in conjunction with the usually recommended exercises for breech or posterior presentation, homeopathic intervention may assist the baby in getting into a favorable birthing position. The program can be started earlier than four weeks if the woman is very short-waisted and baby consistently prefers to be breech or posterior, or later if there is plenty of room and baby's position has been changeable. Even in labor, remedies are worth a try, but chances for success are reduced after the bag of waters has broken or the presenting part has engaged in the pelvis.

First, determine whether there seems to be a normal amount of amniotic fluid around the baby. Too much fluid will keep the baby buoyant and the uterus overextended, so the baby can easily float into an undesirable position. Too little fluid will likewise be problematic as the breech baby will not have enough buoyancy to turn. If fluid levels seem to be off in either direction, try the water-balancing tissue salt **Natrum Muriaticum**. Suggested regimens for varying potencies are as follows (see what works for you):

> 6X 3 times per day for 1 week or
> 30C 2 times per day for 3 days or
> 200C once per day for 3 days or
> 1M once

Choice of potency may depend on what is available to you and how much time you have to work with this problem. Discontinue any dosing if you don't get results or once the baby has turned.

Now, if fluid levels feel normal, then **Pulsatilla** is the remedy of choice and the one that has the most documentation in the homeopathic literature for turning babies. According to Farrington (in his *Clinical Materia Medica*), Pulsatilla acts on the muscular walls of the uterus and stimulates their growth. Sometimes the uterus develops more on one side than another during pregnancy and with this irregularity, the baby assumes an irregular position. Pulsatilla may alter this uneven growth and permit the baby to assume the proper position.

If the woman does not fit the overall Pulsatilla or Natrum Muriaticum symptom pictures, or the baby needs to remain in his/her present position for whatever reason, the remedy may not work. If it does work, it is a most gentle intervention indeed, effecting changes in the baby's environment rather than impacting the baby directly. Definitely worth a try!

Post-Cesarean Regimen

If a situation develops which is beyond the scope of home health care, remedies can be used to help stabilize the person while transport is being accomplished (e.g., Arnica, Aconite, Carbo Veg). Parents and midwives need not be concerned that remedies used at home might interact negatively with drugs or other treatments used at the hospital. Remember, drugs get into the bloodstream but remedies do not. For instance, homeopathic Caulophyllum can be used safely at home to stimulate labor contractions without the risk of lowering the mother's blood pressure associated with full-strength herbal tincture of Blue Cohosh. If Pitocin is later resorted to in a hospital setting, there is no cause for concern. Likewise, during the recovery period, remedies can be used to speed the healing process and reduce or eliminate the need for pain-killing drugs. But mom can also safely take the painkillers if needed. After cesarean section, aggressive use of the following remedies should prove helpful.

Immediately Post-Op

Arnica 200C (1 dose hourly after surgery x3 doses; then

every 3–4 hours for 2 days; follow with Bellis if tenderness, soreness or bruising persists)

Phosphorus 30C (for post-surgical vomiting; repeat after each vomiting episode; or try 1 dose every half hour after surgery x3 doses to help eliminate anesthesia more quickly from the body)

Hypericum 200C (can be given in alternation with Arnica, for pain in the first couple of days post-op)

Staphysagria 200C (1 dose on first day helps expel trapped abdominal gas; can be repeated if gas pains persist; promotes healing of incision site and overall assault on the body)

In a Few Days

Bellis 30C (1 dose daily x3–5 days, after Arnica, if soreness persists)

Calc Fluor 6X (after acute remedies listed above are no longer needed, take 2 tablets twice daily for 2–4 weeks to prevent formation of excessive adhesions and scar tissue)

Calendula 30C (1 dose daily x1 week in cases of poor wound healing)

Staphysagria 200C (1 dose for pain in the incision site)

Administration of Remedies

HOMEOPATHIC REMEDIES SHOULD BE PLACED in the mouth by tapping the correct dosage into the cap and tapping the pellets under the tongue, being careful not to handle the pellets directly or touch the cap to the mouth. Remedies should be administered into a clean mouth with nothing to eat or drink fifteen minutes before and after the remedy is given, but in emergencies don't worry about this. Aromatic oils such as mints (including mint toothpaste), camphor, menthol and oils found in coffee beans should be avoided as they may render the remedies ineffective or antidote one that is working.

I order all of my remedies in the #10 size pellets. These are very tiny sugar pills, about the size of poppy seeds. A few (10–15), equals one dose. They are very easy to administer to babies and are cost effective. Most pharmacies have them, but you will have to specially request them. I don't usually have trouble getting babies to open their mouths for remedies. However, you can also tap a few tiny pellets into the palm of one hand, wet a finger and touch it to the pellets, then allow the baby to suck your finger.

With larger pellets, one can be tapped into your hand and then placed along the inside of the baby's cheek. Don't worry if the baby's tongue thrusting eventually forces the pellet to fall out of the mouth. The healing vibration of the remedy is delivered once it makes contact with the mucous membrane.

Remedies can also be dissolved in water (distilled is ideal, but not necessary) and given to the baby with an eyedropper. It's nice to have a few clean amber glass dropper bottles on hand; either 1/2 ounce or 1 ounce size is fine (see Resources section). If the baby needs more than one trauma remedy, just mix them together in water and give frequently. Such a mixed dosage bottle, for example, might be sent along with the parents for a baby who is transported to the hospital after a homebirth. Parents might claim to curious hospital staff that they are using holy water on their baby, rather than attracting negative attention by being more forthcoming and thereby potentially inviting prejudicial treatment. Or, better yet, just be discreet. Dilutions can be rubbed onto pulse points on the baby if it is impossible to give anything by mouth, but do try to contact the mucous membrane, no matter how miniscule the amount.

Conventional rules surrounding the administration of homeopathic remedies are somewhat mythical. Remedies still work when not placed under the tongue, though the vital force may respond faster if the remedy is placed there. Do be careful not to get saliva on the bottle cap or eyedropper, and refrain from handling the inside rims of the bottles or replacing into the bottle any pellets that may have spilled. The enzymes in saliva or the oils on your hands could contaminate the rest of the remedy in the bottle and render it ineffective. Be sure also not to reuse a bottle for a different remedy, unless it has been sterilized in between.

Legal/Ethical Considerations for Midwives

Be sure to inform your clients, from the beginning of your relationship, that homeopathy is one of the ways that you are prepared to handle complications of labor and delivery. Clarify that you have their consent to do so. Whenever possible, in non-emergent situations, clients should be encouraged to obtain their own remedies. By doing so, you foster a high level of personal responsibility and empower women to access resources on their own. (After all, you don't want to make folks dependent on you, do you?) If you live in an area with limited access to remedies, be aware that most companies listed in the Resources section will Fed Ex remedies overnight.

As homeopathy is not "standard of care" in the United States, be careful about administering remedies to babies or moms when in the presence of emergency medical personnel or hospital staff. You may attract some serious negative attention. Your best protection is to let the parents self-administer. If they are not motivated enough to do so, then you shouldn't be giving remedies in the first place.

Finally, a word of caution about using remedies with women who are threatening a miscarriage. An informed consumer of homeopathy understands that a remedy cannot cause a miscarriage. The remedy simply works *with* the person's vital force, helping it to go in the direction it is already heading to achieve a state of balance. If it is possible to neutralize a trauma or other precipitating cause for a miscarriage (e.g., Aconite or Arnica), the remedy will accomplish that and the pregnancy will hold. However, if the bleeding and cramping are prolonged and a remedy is given, a nonviable pregnancy is likely to be brought to a quick resolution in response. A committed homeopathic patient understands and believes in the benign power of the remedy and is unlikely to second guess the resolution phase, whatever the outcome. However, for someone who may be new to homeopathy, attempting a remedy in this scenario is risky for both the woman and the midwife. The mother's perception may be that the remedy *caused* the miscarriage. And her perception will be her reality. Follow her lead on this and if she needs to hang onto hope, then it may be best to let everything run its own course, unless a need for intervention is clearly indicated. At that point, she can choose the modality she is most comfortable with for treatment.

Dosage Considerations

Dosage refers to both the potency of the remedy chosen and the number of times it is repeated. Many methods of prescribing exist and homeopaths cannot agree upon firm rules or any one system. Following are some general guidelines for midwifery practice.

Low potencies are those below 30C. The most commonly available low potencies are 6X, 12X, 30X, 6C and 12C. The low potencies are often very effective and thought by many to be safer for use by the inexperienced practitioner. High potencies are those above 200C, generally 1M or 10M. The medium potencies, 30C and 200C, are my most common choices in midwifery practice. I have rarely seen an aggravation from them, yet they are strong enough to be effective in most cases.

Prenatally and postpartum, try using a 30C or lower potency repeated three times a day for several days. If there is any positive change, then stick with the remedy, but repeat it only when the action of the last dose seems to have exhausted itself.

Remember, homeopathy does not saturate the blood stream with a medicinal agent (as in herbology or allopathy), but rather imparts a stimulus to the vital force. More is not necessarily better. The ideal dosage is the minimum stimulus a person requires to bring about balance or resolution of symptoms.

If improvement does not commence within a couple of days (or less if the condition is severe), a different remedy can be tried. However, if the remedy seems to help for a day or two and then stops helping, perhaps one dose of a higher potency of the same remedy would be more effective. This is worth a try.

In case an aggravation of symptoms occurs, discontinue the remedy and take a wait-and-see approach. If indeed the remedy did over-stimulate the person and cause a "healing crisis," then, after a brief worsening of symptoms, the person should start to improve. Aggravations can be tricky because it can be difficult to tell whether the person is over-responding to the remedy or the wrong remedy was chosen and they are simply getting worse. There are lots of nuances to homeopathy; it is complex and intricate and it can take years to become truly skilled. The goal is not to stimulate a catharsis (though sometimes that happens). Rather, the gentle cure is what we are after.

During labor and birth, I usually use a 200C potency. If a positive response is elicited, the remedy can be repeated once or twice if the effect begins to wane. However, if no effect is seen after one or two doses, it is assumed to be the wrong remedy and is not repeated.

For conditions that come on suddenly, such as trauma, hemorrhage or a high fever, a 200C or 1M potency may be an appropriate choice. In emergencies, remedies can be repeated every minute or two, depending upon the intensity of the situation. The more emergent the situation, the quicker the expected action of a remedy, so if you don't see results after two doses, try a different remedy.

Infants and small children do not require special consideration regarding dosage. The size of the individual's body is irrelevant. Rather, it is the energy or intensity of the disturbance that one is attempting to match energetically with the dosage. So, for example, if a person has been wasting away from a chronic disease and is in the end stages, low potencies are a better match for the vital force. Sometimes, through trial and error, we learn that a specific person is extremely sensitive to remedies and is therefore better off with low potencies.

How Quickly Should a Person Respond to a Remedy?

Let's go with the image of a bell curve. Each disturbance (discomfort, illness, emergency) has three phases: onset, crisis and resolution. Bell curves comes in different shapes as demonstrated here.

The tall bell curve here shows a sudden onset, short crisis and quick resolution. Think hemorrhage, shock, mastitis with high fever. In these situations, one needs *something* to work *fast*. Amazingly, a correctly chosen remedy will do so and improvement will be rapid—just what is called for (like flipping a light switch—hemorrhage off). The remedy fits the energy of what is happening and moves the person through the course of the disturbance more quickly. If it doesn't work fast, it's not working. With this type of sudden onset or potentially

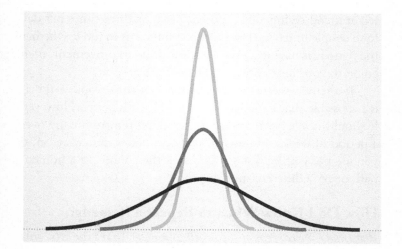

life-threatening emergency, medium and high potencies can be used and repeated every couple of minutes for the first two doses and then another remedy chosen if there is no improvement.

The middle bell curve shows a more common scenario with a short onset, crisis and resolution. Think stalled labor, urinary tract infection, colic. One truly hopes the remedy works, but it is not so urgent. A 30C or 200C remedy might be repeated every couple of hours for two doses and then another chosen if there is no improvement.

Finally, we come to the more flat appearing bell curve. This complaint has come on gradually, slowly getting worse and slowly resolving. Think nausea of early pregnancy, varicose veins, postpartum depression. While less intense overall, it is of longer duration. It is unlikely that the person's response to a well-chosen remedy will be of the dramatic, rapid-improvement-after-one-dose variety. In this situation, I recommend trying a 30C potency two or three times per day for a couple of days. This should be sufficient to judge whether the remedy is having a positive effect. If no improvement, then go on to your next choice and repeat the process.

If a remedy seems to help at first but then stops working, it is possible that a higher potency will work better. However, it should never be necessary to be taking remedies daily over a period of weeks. Homeopathy works better than that. So, if you are not getting results, then seek the counsel of a homeopath or try a different modality.

How Do I Know When to Repeat a Remedy?

Remember the concept of the minimum dose. That's the true rule here. Some homeopathic practitioners prescribe in an allopathic manner (e.g., take three times per day for three days) because people are conditioned to expect specific instructions regarding medications. A more accurate set of instructions involves increased responsibility on the part of the patient (e.g., "repeat the remedy if you are unsure of a response or whenever the person feels worse"). Some folks will simply be too uncomfortable with this. But remember, while we are not attempting to saturate the patient's bloodstream with a medicinal agent as in the case of antibiotics repeated every six or eight hours, this is nevertheless the mindset with which the majority of us are most familiar. If the colic remedy worked last night, it is understandably tempting to want to repeat it tonight in order to "head off" another attack. But really, the remedy should only be repeated when the action of the last dose seems to have worn off and the patient's symptoms are relapsing.

A good metaphor is a child learning to swing on a swing. The parent starts by giving them a push and then another push. Then we back off and let the swing just go. Gradually, the swinging will dwindle to a stop. As it slows down, we step in and give another push. Eventually, the child learns to keep the swing going on their own. No more pushes are needed.

Miscellaneous Topics

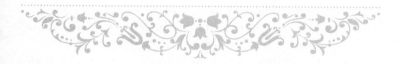

Combination Remedies

Some stores sell homeopathic combination products. The package might say "teething" or "fever" or "colic." This is the shotgun approach to homeopathy. Typically, the top six or so most commonly indicated remedies for teething are mixed together in *very low potency* (1–3X). Often, the combination remedies work because the simillimum (single closest match for the symptom picture) is included and the person resonates with that while the other substances remain dormant. I'm a pragmatist more than a purist and, since a combination remedy might be effective, quick and easy for someone who knows very little about homeopathy, there is no harm in its use. It is, however, a very inelegant and unknowledgeable use of homeopathy and there are some limitations to this practice:

- You have no idea which remedy in the mix the person is responding to. This knowledge might be helpful for more in-depth constitutional treatment by a homeopathic physician. For example, if an infant responds to the colic combination for acute episodes, but continues to experience acute attacks every day, then a more curative remedy should be sought. Since remedies have a relationship with each other, the acute helper remedy may be an important clue to the cure for an experienced homeopath. To understand better which remedy is working in the combination, you could read the symptom picture of each remedy listed on the bottle (see Boericke in the Resources) to see which ones you might eliminate and which is likely the one that is working. Then try a single 30C dose of your top guess and observe the baby.

- In cases where a combination remedy does not work, it is still possible that one of the remedies in that combination is the simillimum but that the person needs it in a higher potency.

- The marketing of these products creates confusion on the part of the consumer regarding what homeopathy is and how it works. The FDA's labeling regulations, in effect, allopath-ize homeopathy. There is no remedy for colic per se; there is only the best match for the symptom picture.

Nosodes

Nosodes are a specific class of remedies that are made from diseased tissues or discharges, for example the sputum of a person suffering from tuberculosis or the discharge of a person suffering from gonorrhea. Admittedly, this is gross, but remember that all remedies contain non-material doses of the natural substance from which they originate. Three nosodes are included in this book: Medorrhinum, Pyrogenium and

Tuberculinum. You may have difficulty purchasing these without a doctor's prescription. Likewise, some pharmacies may not sell high potencies to the lay person (e.g., 1M or higher).

Relationship of Remedies

Just as plants in the garden have "companion plants" or ones that grow particularly well together, so do remedies exhibit a synergistic relationship to each other. In your organic garden, for example, basil and parsley will repel insects that are normally attracted to tomato plants and the trio goes nicely together on the table as well. On the other hand, some plants simply will not grow in proximity to others.

In homeopathy, remedies have been found to have a variety of energetic interactions including complementary (extends or completes the action of, or prepares the way for another remedy), antidotal (cancels the curative action of a remedy if sequenced after it), and inimical (remedies won't work in each other's presence) relationships. Boericke's *Materia Medica With Repertory* (see Resources) is an excellent resource on this subject. Boericke lists the inter-relationship of remedies information under each remedy description and summarizes it in a table in one of the many helpful appendices.

Complementary remedies are always worth considering if you find yourself needing the same acute remedy over and over again. For example, a woman who responds to Nux Vomica for constipation and nausea, but keeps relapsing with her complaints, may need Sepia. Nux is the acute, Sepia the chronic. In the case of PMS, Nux may provide relief when she is in the throws of her PMS, while Sepia in high potency, given after the period is over, may prevent the next month's need for Nux.

Recommended Birth Kit for Midwives

THE FOLLOWING TWENTY REMEDIES fit nicely into a kit for the midwife's birth bag. Over time, as your knowledge and pharmacy grow, you will most likely want to carry with you more of the remedies discussed in this booklet, as well as a variety of potencies of the remedies you use most frequently.

Aconite 200C
Antimonium Tart 200C
Arnica 200C
Arsenicum 200C
Belladonna 200C
Carbo Veg 200C
Caulophyllum 200C
Chamomilla 200C
Cimicifuga 200C
Cinchona 200C

Gelsemium 200C
Hamamelis 200C
Hypericum 200C
Kali Carb 200C
Pulsatilla 200C
Rhus Tox 200C
Sabina 200C
Secale 200C
Sepia 200C
Staphysagria 200C

Bibliography & Resources

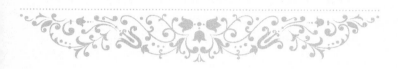

Books

Boericke, William. *Materia Medica with Repertory.* Philadelphia, PA: Boericke & Tafel, Inc., 1927. This is a basic reference book and necessary early purchase for home prescribing.

Brennan, Patty. *Vaccines & Informed Choice: Everything Parents Need to Know, 6th Edition.* Ann Arbor, MI: Dream Street Press, 2015.

Castro, Miranda. *Homeopathy for Pregnancy, Birth, and Your Baby's First Year.* New York: St. Martin's Press, 1992. Good overall resource on the subject. Contains naturopathic options as well as remedy suggestions for common problems.

Coulter, Catherine. *Portraits of Homeopathic Medicines: Psychophysical Analyses of Selected Constitutional Types, Vols. I &II.* St. Louis, MO: Quality Medical Publishing Inc., 1986. Provides in-depth portraits of eighteen important remedies.

Coulter, Catherine. *Portraits of Homeopathic Medicines, Volume III: Expanding Views of the Materia Medica.* St. Louis, MO: Quality Medical Publishing Inc., 1998. This volume is a continuation of her earlier work.

Coulter, Catherine. *Homeopathic Sketches of Children's Types.* St. Louis, MO: Quality Medical Publishing, Inc., 2001.

Hahnemann, Samuel. *Organon of Medicine.* 6th Edition. Pagosa Springs, CO: Hahnemann Academy of North America, 1993. The primary source—a must read.

Herscu, Paul. *The Homeopathic Treatment of Children.* Berkeley, CA: North Atlantic Books, 1991. Modern, user-friendly book helps identify children's constitutional types. Excellent outlines provide a quick summary of each remedy. Coulter gives us the adult version of these remedies; Herscu describes how the remedy pictures manifest in children. Contains a "Notes on Infants" section at the end of each remedy. Excellent reference.

Morrison, Roger. *Desktop Companion to Physical Pathology.* Nevada City, CA: Hahnemann Clinic Publishing, 1998. Contains concise differentials for some of the main pathologies encountered in homeopathic practice. Excellent section on UTIs.

Morrison, Roger. *Desktop Guide to Confirmatory Symptoms.* Albany, CA: Hahnemann Clinic Publishing, 1993. This modern materia medica is one of my favorite clinical aids.

Moskowitz, Richard. *Homeopathic Medicines for Pregnancy & Childbirth.* Berkeley, CA: North Atlantic Books, 1992. Dr. Moskowitz had a homebirth practice and used homeopathy in over 800 pregnancies. His very interesting book contains many case studies with specific dosages reported and an extensive bibliography.

Murphy, Robin. *Homeopathic Medical Repertory: A Modern Alphabetical Repertory, 3rd edition.* Pagosa Springs, CO: Hahnemann Academy of North America, 2005. This repertory was designed to be user-friendly and is. It even contains a section entitled "Pregnancy." I have found it to be extremely clinically helpful.

Panos, Maesimund and Heimlich, Jane. *Homeopathic Medicine at Home.* New York, NY: The Putman Publishing Group, 1980. My favorite beginner's book and resource for acute home prescribing for common first aid crises and acute illnesses.

Shiloh, Jana. *Curing Colic and Lactose Intolerance with Homeopathy.* Sedona, AZ: Rocky Mountain Homeopathics, 1987. This book will clarify where to focus when case-taking for a baby suffering from colic or other digestive difficulties. Helpful charts are user-friendly.

Smith, Trevor. *Homeopathic Medicine for Women: An Alternative Approach to Gynecologic Health Care.* Rochester, VT: Healing Arts Press, 1989. Particularly helpful in the treatment of vaginal infections and breastfeeding difficulties.

The Biochemic Handbook. St. Louis, MO: Formur, Inc., Publishers, 1976. Excellent little book on the use of the homeopathic tissue salts.

Weed, Susun. *Wise Woman Herbal for the Childbearing Year.* Woodstock, NY: Ash Tree Publishing, 1986. Excellent sourcebook on herbal remedies during pregnancy, labor, and postpartum.

Wright-Hubbard, Elizabeth. *A Brief Study Course in Homeopathy.* St. Louis, MO: Formur, Inc., 1977. Describes the homeopath's process in casetaking and choosing a remedy. Good little introductory book.

Resources

Birth With Love Midwifery Supplies
https://birthwithlovestore.com/store/
Homebirth and midwifery supplies, herbs, homeopathics and more.

Boiron-Borneman
http://www.boironusa.com/
Full-service pharmacy and book supplier.

Cascade HealthCare Products, Inc.
http://www.1cascade.com/
Homebirth and midwifery supplies, first-aid items, medical supplies and equipment, books, educational materials, herbs and the recommended homeopathic birthing kit.

Castle Remedies
http://castleremedies.com/
Homeopathic pharmacy, sells the recommended birth kit.

Homeopathic Educational Services
https://www.homeopathic.com/
Book supplier, remedy kits.

Midwifery Supplies Canada
http://www.midwiferysupplies.ca/
Midwifery and doula supplies, first-aid items, books, educational materials, homeopathics and more.

National Center for Homeopathy
http://www.homeopathycenter.org/
Find a homeopath and more.

Natural Health Supply
http://www.a2zhomeopathy.com/
Sells amber glass bottles, including 1/2-dram, 1-dram and 2-dram bottles; also carries dropper bottles (excellent for water dilutions), pellets and plastic cases. Their bottles are a great way to send remedies home with clients or to use in assembling your own kits.

About the Author

OVER 40 YEARS, Patty Brennan has been a doula, midwife, educator, author, nonprofit executive, and entrepreneur. Today, she is the owner of Lifespan Doulas [LifespanDoulas.com], a training company offering professional online doula training and certification for the complete lifespan (birth doulas, postpartum doulas, and end-of-life doulas). Patty has personally trained approximately 2500 people to become doulas. As founder/executive director of two community-based nonprofit doula programs in Michigan, she has helped makes doulas widely available in her home state, especially for low-income families.

Patty became interested in homeopathy after her second son was born in 1985 and experienced multiple chronic health issues through the first year of his life. Through the skillful support of a classical homeopathic physician, her son's afflictions were cured. Patty began to study homeopathy and to integrate the remedies into home health care with her family and homebirth midwifery clients.

Books by Patty Brennan

- *The Doula Business Guide: How to Succeed as a Birth, Postpartum or End-of-Life Doula, 3rd Edition (2019)*
- *The Doula Business Guide Workbook: Tools to Create a Thriving Practice, 3rd Edition (2019)*
- *Guide to Homeopathic Remedies for the Birth Bag, 5th Edition Revised (2022)*
- *Vaccines & Informed Choice: Everything Parents Need to Know, 6th Edition (2016)*
- *Whole Family Recipes: For the Childbearing Year & Beyond (2007)*

All books can be ordered online at www.LifespanDoulas.com. If you live outside of the U.S., I recommend making your purchase on Amazon to save on exorbitant shipping costs. A wholesale discount of 40% is available on orders of 6 or more of any one item.

Made in the USA
Coppell, TX
01 December 2022

87560009R00059